MY BEST FRIEND WAS THE CHOCOLATE CAKE

MY Best friend was THE CHOCOLATE CAKE

Renae Bressi

http://www.overcomeyouremotionaleating.com/

Published by Bubbles & Barefoot Publishing in 2016
First edition; First printing

ISBN 978-0-9945115-0-8

Bubbles and Barefoot Publishing
www.BubblesBarefoot.com

To My loving Mum,

always there, no matter what. Thank you for the sacrifices you've made, the boundless love you give me and the values you have taught me to possess. You have helped shape me into the woman I am today, teaching me every step of the way. Forever grateful for you – I love you xo

My dearest Dad,

you are too beautiful for words. I adore you and feel blessed to have you as my Dad. Thank you for your love, your kindness, your strength and unwavering patience. You mean the world to me and I am eternally grateful that I am your little girl in this life.

My love Damian,

thank you for your endless belief, incredible support and the unquestionable love you give me every day - you have opened my eyes to a part of myself that I want to get to know more of – thank you for coming along for the ride.

And...

the people like me who want more for themselves,

and more from their lives. For the men and women who seek freedom, strive for truth and are ready to take control of their eating habits once and for all. I was once where you are and I know it's possible to be free of emotional eating and live a rich and fulfilling life.

It's a life you deserve.

It's your turn.

Table of Contents

PREFACE

Why I Wrote This Book

I wrote this book for two reasons. Firstly I wrote it to help me heal and secondly I wrote it to help you heal. Two decades of my life were spent emotionally eating. Twenty years. Over half my life. I held onto my secret tightly, so tightly that I didn't allow people or possibilities to enter my space to help me beat my food obsession. Because I built my walls so high, the life I had created for myself was extremely sad, lonely and painful. I thought I was alone and that no one would understand so I kept going on alone, trying to get on top of my emotional eating, without any support. I lived a secret double life where everything appeared wonderful on the outside but on the inside I was struggling day in, day out because I was never able to beat my food 'addiction.'

I used to keep my secret life so close to me that it took a huge amount of energy just to hide it; it was a burden and I would use food as a pick me up which only left me feeling frustrated and defeated because I would regularly overindulge and I would be right back at square one, consumed by negative mind chatter and feeling like a failure.

My past may be behind me now but it is still a part of who I am. Without my experiences I wouldn't be where I am today. The struggles, the pain, the emotional highs and lows, the whole experience, has brought me to this moment and I am stronger for everything I have endured.

Now, I express my emotions in constructive ways, tune into my body and listen to what it really wants and I am more mindful of my triggers. By tuning in, practicing awareness and expressing my emotions constructively, I can get a true reading of what my emotions are trying to tell me and as an added bonus I am able to release built up emotional baggage rather than stuffing my emotions down with food. Food is not the answer, it has never been the answer and will never be the answer and if we listen to our emotions rather than numbing them with food, we will find out what void we are trying to fill with food.

I am honored to do the work I do. It is a privilege to work with other men and women so they too can heal their relationship with food. Together we can heal. It is time to release the burdens we no longer need to be carrying and make room for wonderful things to come into our lives. Letting go of the old, welcomes in the new.

Thank you for reading ❤

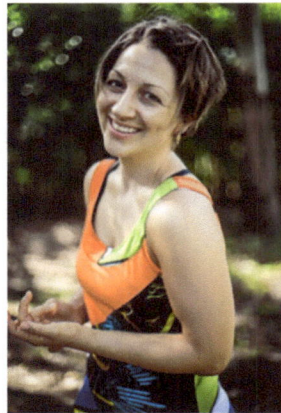

INTRODUCTION

Who Should Read This Book?

This book is for the people out there, who are fed up using food as a crutch. It's for the people, both men and women who lose themselves in food and beat themselves up for doing so. Emotional eating is full of shame, anxiety and despair. As an emotional eater, I was constantly surrounded by negative emotions, feelings of self-loathing, regret and desperation but I always had hope. I knew there had to be an answer and I feel free now that I have found it.

I have a new found freedom and I am here to tell you there is light at the end of the tunnel. You too can be in control of what you eat. I am living proof that it is possible.

I am here to be transparent with you, to let you know that you are not alone, that I too have struggled, that I also have done things behind closed doors that I was so ashamed of and since overcoming emotional eating, I have been able to put those things behind me and accept them as an experience and thanks to that experience, it has given me a whole new perspective on life that I am now able to share with other people, like you. You too can realise you are not alone and that there is hope. I know, because I have made it out the other end of the struggles, turmoil and desperation of being an emotional eater.

And, one more thing. I would just like to say thank you and congratulations for investing in this book and in yourself. I just know that if you take the time and do the work, you too will come out the other side – free of emotional eating.

You've got this beautiful soul,

xo Renae

Chapter One

CONSIDER THIS THE BEGINNING

I love new beginnings. There is nothing like starting something new; whether it be venturing off to a place I have never been, meeting people for the first time, joining a new program or opening a new book. There is something about it that lures me in, makes me want to get in to it and make the most out of it, and the excitement I get is exhilarating.

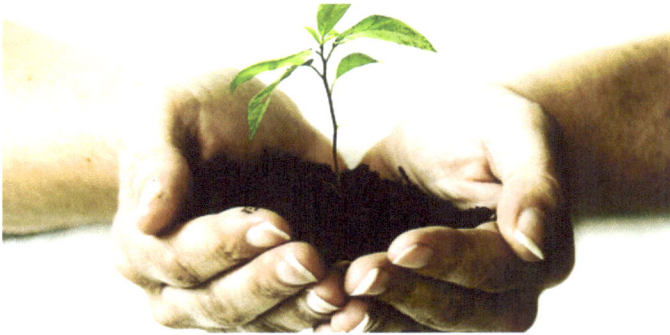

It's like strapping myself in on a freaky rollercoaster – my heart races and I can't wait to see what the new introduction is going to bring to my life. My eyes light up, my voice raises, I become childlike – it takes me back to the excitement I felt when I was young on Christmas eve, when Santa Claus was so close to showering me with my list of gifts that I anticipated receiving – new for me means magical. Do you feel the same or am I alone on this one?

For me, waking up is exciting, I love starting a new day so much that I jump out of bed as early as possible. My alarm rings at 4am, most days and I'm up – I jump up out of bed thanking my lucky stars that I have another day to devour, a day that I can create whichever way I choose. It's mine, mine for the taking and it's up to me how I live it. This is how I always 'thought' life should be. Full of excitement, full of energy and full of whatever I want to include in it. Life: one big game with ups and downs and merry-go-rounds.

But I didn't always feel this way. I went through a large portion of my life low on energy, flat, feeling heavy, lethargic and 'addicted' to food (I will explain the quotation marks later). I was not in control of my life. I let food rule my life. I saw it and I ate it. If it wasn't there, I thought about eating it and if I'd eaten it, I was more times than not, regretting what I ate or how much I ate and hating the constant cycle of Thinking about food – Resisting food – Eating too much food – Feeling full, heavy, bloated and lethargic – then, Nooooooooo! Regretting the Food I practically inhaled! This was my life. It revolved around food or my thoughts around food and I hated it. It got me down, day in day out, night in, night out.

I've always loved food. My mum tells a story of a time when I was just six months old. She had me on her lap at the hospital waiting to get (a shot) immunized. I was laughing at my Nan pulling faces when all of a sudden the Nurse made her way over to her chair and gave me a spoonful of medicine. Without hesitation my mouth opened wide, surrounding the spoon and in the blink of an eye, I pulled my head back hard, removing all the contents offered to me whilst almost removing the spoon from the rather stunned Nurse's hand. I left all three ladies wide eyed, gob smacked and in hysterics. "Wow – she sure likes her food," commented the Nurse.

I was either a born and bred foodie or a little greedy guts right from the moment I popped my head out into the world. Mum always said I was a good eater, meaning, I NEVER left anything on my plate and sometimes I'd finish the leftovers from other people's plates too. What was there was mine for the taking and even though I was a shy kid, I wasn't shy to take my massive share of food.

Mum never gave my brother and I junk food when we were really young. She said that when we started to get invites to birthday parties was when she lost all control of what we ate and how much we ate… and so did I. I loved going to parties, I loved them so much that I even managed to weasel my way into my older brother's friends' parties. Apparently, I'd look sad when we went to drop him off and for that reason I'd get an invite too – Score!

I especially loved it when Mum would throw my brother and I a party because she always wanted to give us the best birthday party possible, and that she did. There were balloons galore, loads of games and the food was everything a child could possibly want. All those mixed lollies, the assorted chocolates, the fairy bread, toffees, cupcakes, chocolate crackles, party pies drowned in my beloved tomato sauce, red cordial and of course the birthday cake, made with love by Mum with the recipes courtesy of 'The Australian Women's Weekly Children's Birthday Cake Book'. All the typical party staples.

We weren't aware of how to make children's birthday parties healthy back then (and still keep children happy). Not like now, where we can get children eating healthy with so many healthy alternatives around that look and taste good and they are much welcomed, especially due to the rise and rise of allergies in children these days. There is also an array of raw dessert recipes that really do compare taste-wise to the highly processed desserts I grew up on. I don't know how parents managed to control their children after those hyped up birthday parties. We were walking, talking sugar highs.

I recall a party that I went to when I was about six years old where I had seriously abused food. I went crazy with everything that was on offer and before the party had even finished, I had paid dearly for my over the top stuffing-fest. It was coming to the end of the afternoon and parents were starting to arrive to pick up their children. Mum and Dad were going to arrive shortly but I felt really sick and swiftly made my way to the only bathroom in the house where I became a human Vomatron. The sink was my savior and thank goodness I made it. But wait… there's more. I was repeatedly sick in that sink, and not only was I sick, I felt very sorry for myself. I ran the tap so the mess would go down the sink. I needed to wash away all the evidence, but Noooooo, the chunks wouldn't go down, in fact, I had completely blocked the sink and there was an embarrassing pile of mess before me. There was a knock at the door. "Renae, are you in there? Mrs Cass called, your parents are here." Oh, no, I couldn't believe this was happening. I tried to drown the evidence but to no avail. "Renae, your Mum and Dad are waiting." I was mortified. "I'm coming!" There was nothing more I could do. I had to leave the bathroom and face the parents.

Because I was such a shy kid, confessing to what had happened wasn't an option, I never would've been able to look Mrs Cass in the eye and tell her what had happened. So, I didn't. I walked out of the bathroom, closing the door behind me while looking as confident as possible to give the impression that nothing out of the ordinary had happened while I was in the bathroom. When I was taken to my parents, I thanked my host and left without saying a word about the sink that was full of regurgitated party food. Oh, the shame!

I never found out what happened regarding the sink incident, I'm not sure if they knew it was me or if it remained a mystery in that house for years, all I know is that I didn't learn my lesson and continued to over indulge in food.

When I reached high school, I had what was described by some of my friends a 'fascinating way of eating'. That's what they said to my face, I'm not sure how they described it behind my back. I'm sure it wasn't worded as socially acceptable as 'fascinating' when I wasn't around and I can't blame them. Let me give you an example. When I went to McDonalds in my teens I would never just order and eat. I used to play around, invent new meals and mix my ingredients. I'd remove the bottom part of the bun from my Big Mac (I thought it was bland. I didn't do bland) and I'd flip the burger over, spread a packet of sweet and sour sauce all over the bottom, which now became the top and I'd bite into the upside down burger and get sauce all over my top lip and my fingers would get all sticky as I bit down into the burger, making a mess of my meal. The fries got dipped in soft serve and sometimes the nuggets would get a turn of being covered in ice-cream too. I'm sure it turned people off but I didn't enjoy McDonalds any other way. I only liked the reinvented version.

Buffets were my favourite because I could mix and match everything and I never left the restaurant without being choc-a-block stuffed… and I thought it was normal to do that.

I was an overeater well into my early thirties, much to my own disapproval. But what's a girl to do if she doesn't know any other way to deal with situations? I'll tell you what she does, she continues to eat, bottling up her feelings and numbing her pain with food… food, glorious food – oh, the irony.

I am often asked if I was ever overweight as a child because of the amount of food and junk food I ate. The answer is no, I was never overweight as a child and all of my friends would probably say that I was never overweight in my teens but I beg to differ.

Throughout primary school I was lucky in the fact that even though I ate a tonne of garbage, my weight never changed, which I thought was fantastic because I could eat whatever I wanted, whenever I wanted. Aside from the meals Mum would make at home (which I normally had a second helping of) I ate a lot of junk food, but I never had to worry about putting on kilos, so putting on weight was a non-issue for me back then. In fact, I thought that was the only reason we shouldn't eat junk food (because you'd put on weight) but that never happened to me so there was no reason for me to stop eating CRAP.

C - Carbonated Drinks

R - Refined Sugars

A - Artificial Sweeteners and Artificial Colours

P - Processed Foods

On my walk to school with friends, we'd stop and get some sweet treats to get us through the day. We'd stock up on lollies, chocolates, two minute noodles with spicy seasoning, fruit juice or soft drink and I always had a packet of chips at hand, and it was almost always a packet of my beloved salt-n-vinegar. Ahhh how I remember those days. If I had a packet of salt-n-vinegar chips, everything was A-OK.

I didn't develop a real complex around my weight until my early teens and I would judge and criticise my body constantly. I thought my thighs were too big, my face was too round and my breasts weren't the right shape or size. I thought, if only I were a little thinner, then I'd be more popular or if only I had space between my thighs (now known as the 'thigh gap') I'd be more attractive. Yep, I embraced the good for nothing 'If only' syndrome. I played the victim. I'd think why me, why can't I look like her – her being the most popular girl in school. I spent a lot of time wishing I looked like someone else, wishing I was someone else, wishing for something that appeared to be better than what I had.

It wasn't until I turned 17 that I was really given something to complain about. I gained seven kilos almost overnight. Now I really thought I was fat. All the poor food choices, starvation diets and binge eating sessions had taken their toll and my self-sabotage (all the abuse I'd been dishing out on myself throughout the years) had finally caught up on me. I *really* started to hate my body when the weight piled on, and it was time for drastic measures. I'd avoid food for up to a week at a time, only allowing myself diet soft drinks and the occasional snack just so I could fit into my skinny jeans for a school dance. I'd have a great time as the thin chick and as a bonus I'd fill my empty tank with all the compliments from friends about how good I looked and then, when my mission was complete, I'd go back to eating my beloved chips and chocolate (because I couldn't take the deprivation anymore) and put the weight back on again within hours. This went on for years. There was so much deprivation, so much gluttony, and so much confusion around food and what it took to be thin. I did what I knew to get thin, inspired by reading gossip magazines but never talked about the measures I took to lose weight… with anyone. I was far too embarrassed about what I was doing. I wore a mask and it was plastered on.

I worked in a newsagency throughout my teenage years and had unlimited access to the latest fashion magazines. I would be sure to get my monthly Girlfriend and Dolly fix and I would look through the glossy magazines from France and the weekly women's 'bibles', so I was never short of getting a peek of that unobtainable magazine photoshopped beauty.

Those magazines helped shape my opinions. I thought women were supposed to be thin and gorgeous and perfect to look at. I thought that's what made you happy and popular and that's what got you a boyfriend and kept him around.

I was in a constant battle with myself to be picture perfect. Little did I know those pictures weren't real. I didn't know they'd been touched up, altered and refined to sell us on a non-truth. I was striving for the impossible. I'd try to reach what didn't exist and I'd come crashing down, reaching out for a quick pick-me-up to ease the disappointment. It didn't help that I worked behind a counter of sweets, a shelf of chocolate, a chip stand and a drink machine and without exaggeration I would say that no less than half of my weekly pay would be spent on junk food. It was there. I could have it, so I did.

My bosses loved the sweet treats too and so did their children. It was acceptable to eat junk food every day. It was the norm. We thought back then that the only thing that was bad about junk food was that it made you fat and I was repeatedly told that I had nothing to worry about because I was young and energetic, so I would burn the calories. So my beliefs were in constant conflict.

STOMACH PAINS

I used to get stomach pains from a very young age. I was in primary school when they started. They were quite regular and I remember that I would hold my stomach regularly to try and ease the pain. I was a Cross Country runner at school and I would put it down to that, thinking that I ran too hard, hence the pain. One day I remember my Mum taking me to the Pathologist to get a blood test. They took what *seemed like all* my blood and despite my large donation, there was no evidence of anything wrong with me when the results came back.

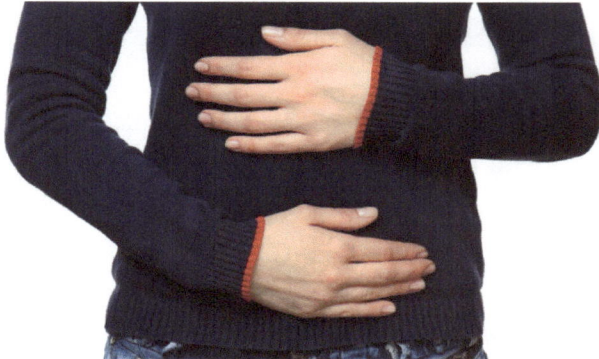

I overheard my Mum telling my Dad that she suspected my beloved salt n' vinegar chips to be the culprit because that was what I ate a lot of. When I overheard this, I never complained about stomach pains again because I thought my parents would do something drastic... ban me from eating chips. Now, that would have been the worst thing that could've happened back then, even worse than if I had been told I couldn't play with my best friend, (now how's that for poor priorities?) so I stayed quiet and endured stomach pains for over half my life. I just dealt with it, got used to it and eventually accepted it as normal and did nothing to change those circumstances... except eventually giving up Cross Country. Isn't it interesting what we accept as normal because we don't want to go through a different kind of discomfort? Instead of tuning into our bodies we tune out with food.

Our bodies are designed to feel... energised, vital and enlivened. All it takes is for us to show up and be ready to change.

HIDING FOOD

When Mum bought treats they wouldn't last long because they would be eaten as if they were a meal. My Dad never had a sweet tooth; it was my Mum, my brother and I who would demolish the sweet stuff. I used to get a hold of it, take my share and put some away for a rainy day, the rainy day usually being over the next couple of days. I always had some kind of treat hidden away somewhere and this continued throughout my life. If there was nothing in the pantry at the time my Mum or my brother wanted a sweet fix, they would come to me because they knew I had the goods. I was like a drug dealer; people would come to me when they wanted their fix. Sometimes I would share if I could see they really *needed* it, unless I didn't have enough rations to go round.

I continued to hide food when I moved out of home. I always had a secret stash of treats around the house. I had numerous hiding spots and when I would indulge and eliminate one secret stash; there were generally others that awaited my next binge. My treats would help me deal with my boredom, sadness, frustration and my loneliness. They were always there for me, to keep me company and help me get through my uncomfortable feelings, and that discomfort was always relieved... but only until the next bite.

By hiding food I felt sneaky because I always had a secret no one knew about. It was a secret I thought I would never share because I didn't think this was something other people did and I was ashamed that I did it. I thought I was the only one or at the very least, I didn't really think about it because I was so consumed with my own food obsession that I didn't think too hard about what was happening in other people's worlds. The reality I have found is that other people are no different from me as this is a very common problem in society. People are just too afraid to speak up and ask for help because like me they fear judgment or lack belief that they too can overcome emotional eating. Or, it could just be they are not quite ready to stop treating food as a friend... yet.

I was also too afraid to speak up for all those reasons but I am so glad I did because my life has completely changed since tackling this challenge. By admitting I had a problem and asking for help I have not only found a way to overcome emotional eating, I have also found a way to help others help themselves and that is the most wonderful gift I can give. Being able to give back makes everything I have gone through a complete blessing.

DIETS WITH MY FRIENDS

In high school I was encouraged (without any persuasion) to go on diets because my friends also wanted to lose a few kilos. There were so many of us girls (and guys) that wanted to be thinner in high school and that desire continued when I went out into the work force. It was never any different, in fact, wherever I went; every new job I was in, every country I visited, there were a large number of us girls (and some guys) and eventually women (and men) who wanted to lose weight. When we complained about one body part or another or when one of the girls wanted to drop, sometimes over 10 kilos, we would always think each other was crazy but when it came to ourselves, we thought we were fat. I find it interesting that we loved each other no matter what shape or size we were but we just couldn't accept ourselves for what we had and who we were. So, we'd set a date to get to our dream weight; it was always a Monday that we'd start our restriction. We'd plan what we were allowed to eat. On the menu there would be a bowl of cereal for breakfast, a salad sandwich for lunch, a Caramello Koala as a snack (chocolate always showed up at some point in my 'diet') and whatever Mum made for dinner. Usually a bowl of pasta or meat and three veg (without the second helping). Some of us lasted longer than others (or so we told each other) but generally we would never last longer than a week and sooner rather than later I'd be enjoying a bag of chips and a block of chocolate by the weekend, right after I decided that I didn't need to go on a diet after all. Pretty soon I'd eat so much that I was full, bloated and sick and I'd be telling myself I should start another diet… on Monday. Every one of us would play our lack of self-control down, laughing it off as if it didn't really matter… but, it did. It did to me anyway, because behind closed doors I was miserable. My smile came out when I was out in public but it was another story when I was alone. I wasn't coping well and for that reason my food and emotional issues went on for years and they did with my friends too. Some of my friends went on to struggle with anorexia, battle with bulimia, others with obesity, emotional eating, depression and that doesn't happen if you are living a happy, healthy and fulfilling life. I went through the same unhappiness as my friends and I didn't know what to do to stop the insanity, so I ate. I couldn't control myself. I was a slave to my food 'addiction' and that instant gratification was a stronger driver than the long term goal.

THE BINGE EATING DISORDER

The binge eating disorder involves eating large amounts of food frequently and experiencing an inability to stop eating even when we are physically full. Although a good number of people overeat on special occasions; such as birthdays, weddings, holidays, anniversaries, celebrations, Sundays etc., some people overeat excessively and are out of control and this gradually becomes a regular habit. This is known as binge eating.

When you have a binge eating disorder, you may after some time associate too much pain with eating too much and consciously decide to stop. You could however be faced with strong urges to eat that are difficult to resist and thereby continue binge eating. This is what happened to me.

I would eat until I was uncomfortably full. Pasta was a food I would overindulge in and I would do it regularly because it was served regularly in my household growing up. My Dad is Italian and Italian families eat a lot of pasta. I loved that we ate pasta several times a week, I loved pasta so much that ten times out of ten, I would overindulge; sometimes I would go for seconds, sometimes thirds but it wouldn't matter because I knew a way to make my stomach go down after every meal where I had overeaten.

My friend came over one afternoon after school and during this visit, she taught me what she'd learnt at school from her friends. Apparently all the girls were doing it. It was a way to keep your weight down and it allowed you to eat whatever you wanted. I was intrigued, could this really be true? I listened. The technique involved putting your fingers down your throat and purging. It was a hit with me and I started using this technique from that day on. I had to get the method down pat because some foods didn't come up too well, especially if I hadn't had a heap of liquid in the process. I soon caught on and this became my preferred method for keeping my weight down. What's crazy is how delusional I was because I never really lost any body fat, only fluid but I was still happy about seeing fewer kilos on the scales. If the scales showed I weighed a couple of kilos less than the day before, this was a good day, but I would always be up and down (depending on the day) so this method clearly didn't work. I would lose some fluid here and there but my body fat remained the same, but I still thought this was great because the scales told me I was lighter than the day before.

I knew I had a problem when I started taking laxatives. I used to get them from the chemist, making out they were for my Nanna and I would overdose until I had gone too far. Sometimes I would take ten laxatives at a time and I really suffered when I took it that far. It was the most horrible, painful feeling I could imagine at the time and every time I was sitting on the toilet feeling like death, I would ask myself, why? Why am I doing this to myself? And I would then make a promise to myself, every time not to do it again but that was a lie. I would overindulge in food again and again and put myself through the ringer repeatedly. And I wasn't even fat! Sure I weighed a few extra kilos than I wanted to but my obsession to be thin made me go to some ridiculous and punishing extremes. Laxatives were taken in really 'extreme' cases, when I was trying to get thin for a special occasion or if my pants were starting to feel way too tight.

I don't recall taking laxatives too often as it was such a painful experience and because I had read horror stories about people ruining their bowel movements from abusing these pills, besides the fact that it was embarrassing buying them at the chemist, it was such a terrible experience that I didn't like reliving that scenario too often. I read about some girls taking 100 laxatives in a day and couldn't fathom the horrible experiences they would've gone through to get to that number of laxatives in the first place. The pain they would've endured is terrifying. I can only imagine the amount of encounters of excruciating pain they went through to build up to that number of pills. I was in shock that people went to that kind of extreme and my heart went out to them. I was only a tenth of where they were at, so I would tell myself that it wasn't that bad and that there were people worse off than me.

I think about this statement now and it's the reason I write this book. For years I was too embarrassed to talk about this issue, I thought I would be judged. I thought that if I could get past this then I would never have to speak about all of these experiences that I went through…ever. I thought I could just bury this part of my life and pretend to be the person I was pretending to be and no one would be any wiser. This is not the person I choose to be anymore. I want to tell people that I've been there, that I understand; that I get overeating.

I get sitting around for hours eating everything that takes your fancy.

I get being drawn to chocolate bars daily. I get binging and purging.

I get staying at home because you ate too much and feel and look too bloated to go out with your friends.

I get saying "Today is the day I'm going to start this detox and in two weeks I'll have everything under control."

I get "I can't stop."

I get "I need help."

I get feeling like no one else gets it. I get opening the fridge or pantry ten times in an hour.

I get eating one biscuit and before you know it the packet is gone.

I get finishing a binge and promising yourself that was the last time you will do it.

I get the self-loathing and the despair.

I get it, I've been there. I was an emotional eater for more than half my life and I would binge and purge for the best part of twenty years, and although your story will be different to mine, I still know what you are going through. Emotional eaters: we think that no one will get it, that we would be judged, that people would think less of us and that no one understands because they have never walked a mile in our shoes so we keep it a secret; our little secret.

You might think that what people don't know won't hurt them; or you might feel you're not ready to give this up yet, that you don't know of any other way so you listen to your mind and decide to keep it to yourself, and that's ok. You don't have to go out and shout it to the world; I'm not saying that at all. All I'm saying is that I get it. It wasn't easy for me to get to this point and it all started with me confiding in one person that I trusted with all my heart, and then another. Then I was brave enough to get coaching around this, and then I spoke in front of groups because I was sick of pretending to be something I wasn't, pretending that I had everything worked out and that life was peachy. People thought I was healthy and fit because I train at the gym regularly, do yoga, eat well in public and smile a lot. The truth however, was that I was being eaten up inside and it was time to come clean and be free and real and it was time to open the conversation. I needed to let others know that it's ok to not be ok and.... in the process, let go of thinking that I would be judged severely. What people think of me is none of my business.

People will think what they like, when they like, and if I let that stop me from being me, then that's a life half lived; a life lived in fear, a life of holding back, always just giving short of one hundred per cent.

I love the quote from the Bible that goes a little like this "Let he who is without sin, cast the first stone." (And even if you have never read the Bible, it still makes sense to take this quote on board, because it applies to us all). This quote helped me let go of judgment. Like it or not, everyone has done something that can be judged, yes, everyone. None of us are innocent so why do we continue to hide and pretend that we are the one who is perfect? The only judgment we have to let go of is the judgment we have of ourselves. It is then that we can be truly free.

ANOREXIA AND BULIMIA

A study carried out by the Australian Institute for Health and Welfare states more than a million Australians are suffering from some form of eating disorder (Anorexia, Bulimia, Binge Eating or Eating Disorder Not Otherwise Specified); and nearly two-thirds of them are women. In 2012 alone, these disorders resulted in over 1,800 deaths. That's just over 34 deaths a week. *

People with Anorexia are afraid of gaining weight and have a distorted image of their body size and shape. Therefore, they consume very small amounts of food. Most people with Anorexia are underweight. This is because they restrict their food intake through dieting, exercise and fasting. They eat very little for the fear of eating too many calories.

On the other hand, there are people with Anorexia that also binge eat and purge. They eat lots of food and then try to get rid of the calories by making themselves throw up, expelling waste through the aid of diuretics, laxatives and enemas or participating in excessive exercise and crash diets to make up for a binge.

Bulimia is similar to Anorexia in the fact that both sufferers want to be thin. People who have Bulimia may binge eat and then make themselves vomit to prevent weight gain. Repeating this on a long term basis can be very dangerous to a person's health, leading to compulsive behaviors that can be hard to stop. People who suffer from Bulimia, binge and purge on a regular basis, at least once a week for months, even years. They eat large amounts of food (mostly junk food) in one sitting, sometimes in hiding. Some even go to the extent of eating uncooked and frozen foods. They feel powerless to stop eating and can only do so when there is no more space in their stomach for food.

The major difference between people having Anorexia and Bulimia is that those with Anorexia are usually underweight and thin, whereas those with Bulimia can have average weight or be overweight.

I was always intrigued by different forms of eating disorders, probably because I would bounce between them. I would come across articles and read them, word by word, wondering why people would do this to themselves, all the while wondering why I would do it to myself. I think my intrigue was really about wanting to know the reason why I did this so I could cure myself then and there, and never have to tell a soul. I wondered why I starved myself and why I binged and purged. I wanted an answer but I was too afraid to talk to someone about it because I thought that I would be 'taken away' or constantly watched or even worse, force-fed. I would justify my not telling anyone by believing others were in a worse situation than me because they'd been found out; because they couldn't hide it anymore as they were too thin or were caught throwing up. I always thought that I would be ok too, that I could stop anytime. That's what I would repeatedly tell myself. 'I have it under control'.

Back in the 90's I was intrigued by the story of the Kendall Twins, the young sisters who lost their battle with Anorexia and their lives. They were skeleton-thin. Michaela was the first to die at 30 years old, weighing in at less than five stone. Her body was stick thin resembling a starved concentration camp prisoner. Her sister, Samantha took her own life a few years later because of Anorexia and partly because she missed her sister so much that she didn't have the will to go on anymore without her. I wondered what could take people to this extreme – starving themselves to death and thinking that they were fat when clearly they were extremely thin.

Chapter Two

WILLPOWER

WHY IT DOESN'T WORK

What Is Willpower? Willpower as defined by the American Psychological Association is 'the ability to resist short-term temptation in order to meet long-term goals'.

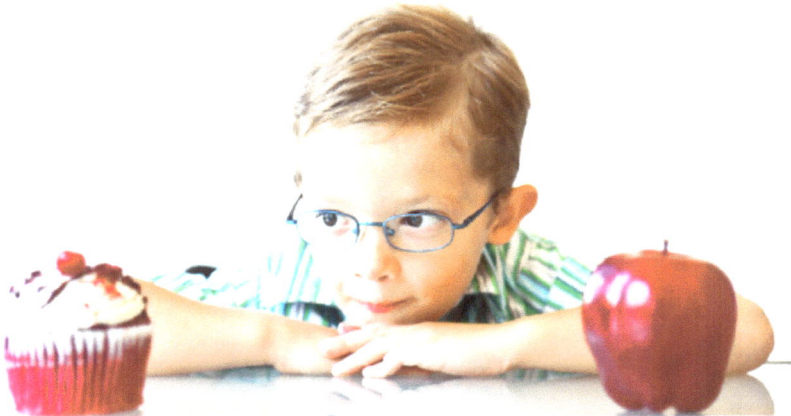

But does willpower work for weight loss and emotional eaters? How many times can an emotional eater resist temptation before giving in to it? Once, twice, ten times? Is it really willpower at play here or does one simply start working through their challenges to change their lifestyle and become the person they really want to be?

Willpower can be used to delay gratification. For example, deciding to skip that second slice of cake you really want or deciding to postpone buying something that wasn't in your budget. It can be about taking positive action, like working out as you had planned, even if you really don't feel like it.

Willpower is a great skill to have, but it is a short-term skill. You will achieve tremendous results if you use it for things like studying for exams or for other short term goals. This is because you may not have enough power to sustain it for a long time. People run out of will power, they run out of the ability to deprive themselves. Therefore, willpower will not work for weight loss, which is a long term goal.

Long-time eating researcher Traci Mann made it known in an interview that willpower does not work for weight loss. She spent more than 20 years studying how people eat and she discovered that willpower does not work the way people imagine it to. The body is predisposed to maintain a weight that does not seem to fit the ideal mould people desire to achieve.

In a study carried out on willpower and weight loss, participants were asked to fill out surveys measuring their willpower as they were offered chips but discouraged from eating them. The participants who indicated they had more willpower on the survey were no less likely to eat the chips.

This research negates the assumption of fat people being lazy and weak-willed while thin people are strong and determined, and proves it to be a myth. You may have a great deal of willpower but still find it difficult to resist your cravings. Scientists concluded that no matter how hard you try to control what you eat using willpower, you will constantly be reminded to eat as food is necessary for our survival.[*]

I spent years living in frustration, feeling as if I was banging my head up against a wall and I just kept going around in the same vicious cycle of:

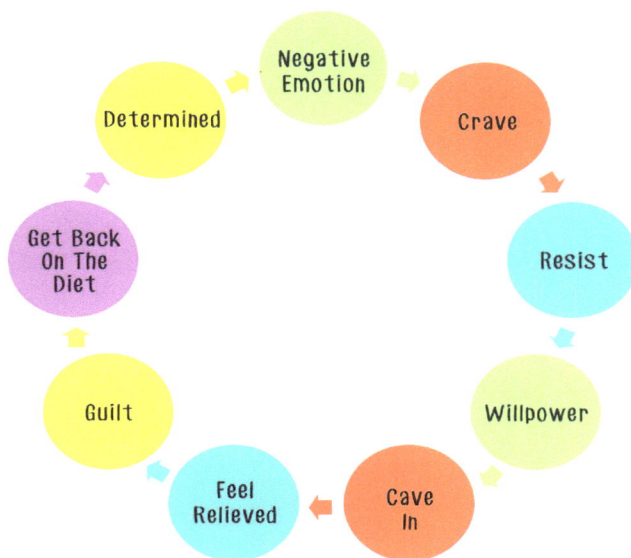

Negative Emotion

Determined

Crave

Get Back On The Diet

Resist

Guilt

Willpower

Feel Relieved

Cave In

I would be feeling determined and in control one day, then totally out of control and low on self-esteem the next day. There were so many ups and downs and more often than not, I felt like I was going backwards more so than forwards. I would take two steps forward and before I knew it I'd taken four giant steps back. I couldn't understand why I was unable to get my eating habits on track. I was so confused at my 'lack of willpower'. I constantly asked myself why I craved chocolate bars every day and why I was unable to go more than a few hours without thinking about where my next meal was coming from. I was forever resisting the urge to eat, and then caving in after a short time of resistance. I was baffled by what was going on. I honestly thought that if I had enough willpower over the course of a few weeks, my 'addiction' would disappear into the abyss and then and only then would I be able to live a life free of wanting the sweet and salty stuff.

What I found after years of frustration and thinking that I was weak was that willpower doesn't work and here's why....

It's generally making a decision from frustration – you think, "right, I'm going on a diet. I don't want to be fat! I'm going to get fit and healthy" without knowing the real reason why.

When there is no firm "why" behind why we want to lose weight or get healthy, we are not heading towards anything, instead we are trying to get away from something with no clear goal 'reward' in sight. This feels like punishment and restriction and because of this harsh approach, we can only hold out for so long.

A better approach would be, really understanding the reason behind why you want to gain control over your eating habits, why you want to lose weight, why you want to get healthy. What is this going to give you? How will you feel when you get your goal? When we dig deep and find the real reason and that reason is strong enough and the feeling it is going to give us is instilled within us, we can then use techniques that are longer lived than using willpower.

A technique that has helped me immensely is:

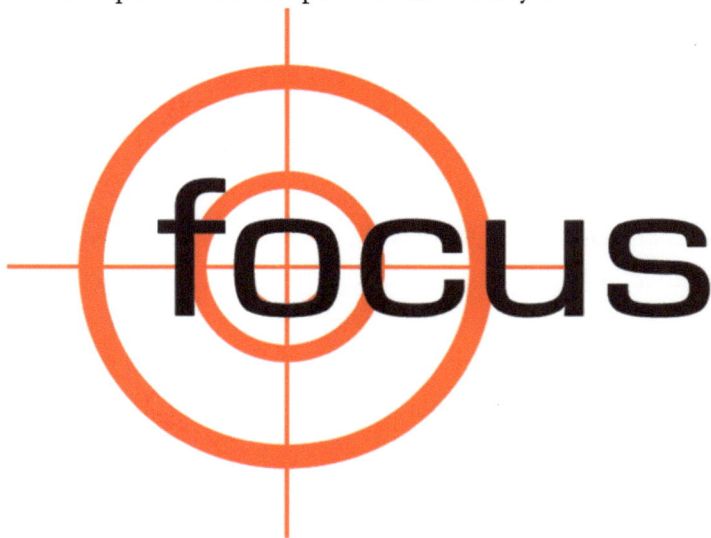

focus

Focus On Your Life

We spend so much time focusing on what we eat rather than why we eat. I've seen people questioning whether they can eat certain foods time and time again on diet sites. Asking questions such as, 'Can I have some tomato with this lunch plan?' 'Am I allowed to eat a piece of meat?' Grown adults asking permission to eat certain foods as if we were children. I use 'we' because I used to do the same. I would cut out a teaspoon of butter to cut down on calories and fat intake. I would be so careful with my portion control and meal planning but I would give into my chocolate bar craving and dive into some chips because I couldn't take the over-abused control anymore. What I was doing was truly unsustainable.

It was exhausting and although it seemed like I was in control (at times) my emotions were controlling me. When I was out at lunch with friends I would just order a salad and they'd think, wow, you're so good, you eat so well but behind closed doors, there was another side, a side that I wasn't showing the world.

After years of going round and round in circles I discovered something that left me gob-smacked. It involved shifting my focus.

I had always wanted to start my own business but I was unsure what I wanted to do. I thought university might help me make a decision. So I went to university and did a Communications Degree – majoring in Marketing and Public Relations. It was ok. It didn't excite me though. It wasn't until I discovered Coaching; with two years remaining in my Bachelor's that marketing got me excited because I was able to understand why we are so drawn to foods. The answer was in our emotions. Marketers base their advertising on emotions. Why? Because people buy on emotion.

Once you are in, they've got you because you then have an emotional attachment to certain foods. If you are connected to something emotionally - you don't stand a chance. It made me think back to the Smith's "Chippie Chippie Chippie" advertisement that featured the Gobbledok that I used to watch when I was a child. I was sold on those chips even before I went to school, plus my Mum was hooked as well so it wasn't hard to get access to these emotional saviors.

I'll explain more about this connection when I speak about the 6 core human needs.

As I had been emotionally attached for so long to certain foods, I had some work to do from the inside out. It was time to understand the real reason behind why I ate those chips daily and this led me to our core human needs.

Chapter Three

THE 6 CORE HUMAN NEEDS – AND HOW
THEY RELATE TO EMOTIONAL EATING

We all have needs in life and yes, food is one of those needs but constantly thinking about food, reaching for highly processed, non-nutritious food is not a need, it's a want. And it's a want that we crave because there are needs; important needs that we need to fill in our life. Our souls have needs, they crave those needs and if your subconscious mind and soul have to get a need fulfilled, they are going to get it fulfilled in whatever way they know how.

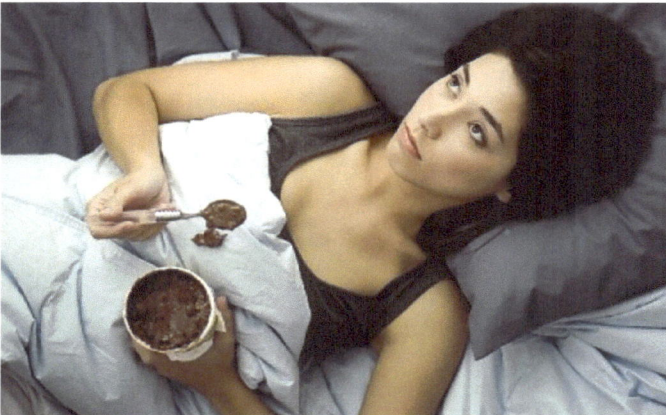

Some people turn to drugs to get their needs fulfilled, other people will turn to alcohol to fulfil their needs and emotional eaters turn to food and the food then becomes a crutch in order to fulfil a deeper need in their soul.

If you eat for reasons other than hunger, you are doing so to fulfil a need that is not being met in constructive ways.

This will become clearer as I go into detail about the universal needs of the soul.

There are 6 essential needs that our souls crave. These needs were coined as 'The 6 Core Human Needs' by the one and only, Tony Robbins. Through learning about and studying these needs, I've been able to have a greater understanding of how to work towards my goals, and my most rewarding so far… Overcoming Emotional Eating. Cheers to that!

The 6 Core Human Needs are as follows:

1. Certainty
2. Variety
3. Significance
4. Love and Connection
5. Growth
6. Contribution

Needs 1 to 4 are personality needs, we need to fulfil these needs for a good life, which is ok but therein lies the issue. If we are living a good life, a safe life, a life that keeps us comfortable in our comfort zone, it stops us from stepping up because things are good (or at least ok). We are snug and cosy and we don't want to take a risk just in case it all goes pear shaped.

Have you ever heard of the term 'Good is the enemy of Great?' You see most of us live a good life which stops us from moving out of our comfort zone, which prevents us from living a great life: Fear sets in… "What if I take this risk and lose it all; what if I become highly successful and lose my circle of friends; what if I speak up and say how I really feel or tell people what's really going on and I am ridiculed?" Do any of these questions sound familiar?

Generally, and I am speaking generally here, we are afraid to live a great life. It's not that we don't want to, it's just that too much is at stake. So, we stop at meeting the first 4 needs (and oftentimes we don't even meet all of those constructively) BUT…

A great life awaits us when we fulfil needs 5 and 6 too. These are the spiritual needs, the needs that really make our soul sing. Get these needs met in constructive ways and you will not only live a good life, you'll live a great life, a fulfilled life. Needs 5 and 6 is where the magic happens.

Take note: If just *one* of the first 4 needs isn't met constructively, (and instead is met unconstructively), it will then show up in the form of an addiction and like I mentioned earlier, emotional eaters will turn to food to fill that need. So as you can see, it is not your fault. You are doing what you can to fulfil that need. It's the way you know, and you know it well. It has worked in the past and continues to work now, even though you are constantly beating yourself up over it, because for a brief moment that need is being met with food.

Interesting, don't you think?

Let me explain this for you need by need so you can understand the needs that you've been filling unintentionally.

1. Certainty

This is the need to feel safe and secure. We need to feel as if we're not under threat of any kind, as if there's no lack of anything; that we have all our basic needs provided. We have food, water, shelter, a stable job and a steady income so we can pay all our bills. We also need to feel that we have stable relationships and that our partner is always going to be there for us; that they're not just going to up and leave us. So most of us have this need met when we're children because our parents or our guardians provide everything for us. They provide our food, water and shelter. They're the ones with the job and the income so they take care of all the bills, we don't even need to think about those and Mum and Dad are always there to protect us and take care of us. So generally, for most of us, we have certainty in our lives when we're children.

Now, when I was a child, I ate a lot of salt and vinegar chips. I had a lot of certainty in my life as a child and I ate a lot of salt and vinegar chips so my subconscious mind had made the connection between certainty and salt and vinegar chips.

Fast forward 20 years, whenever I was having any relationship dramas or any money struggles, whenever my life was in any chaos, stress or bedlam I would instantly reach for the salt and vinegar chips.

I spent so much time, money and energy trying to get over my chip 'addiction' and what I realise now is that I wasn't addicted to the chips, it was the certainty I was reaching out for. So the way I overcame my chip addiction, was by doing some work on myself and realising that I don't need anything external in my life to provide me with certainty, I have it all within me and I'm not talking about just thinking it, I'm talking about deeply feeling it.

2. VARIETY

This is all about diversity, change, new stimuli. If there's not enough excitement in our lives, emotional eaters will turn to food to find that excitement.

Now this excitement personally came through chocolate bars. I thought chocolate was the most exciting thing around. There was a time I was living a very boring, very mundane life. I was working in a job I really didn't like, I was studying at University doing a degree that I didn't really love – the main reason I went to University was to get out of a job that was crushing my soul, but I had no real direction. And here's the topper I was living with my ex-boyfriend who was also my ex-boyfriend at the time so I had to be careful around him so I didn't push any of his buttons. So, just to recap – working in a job I really didn't like, coming home and doing University assignments – tip-toeing around the ex-boyfriend so I didn't ruffle any feathers. As you can probably imagine, life was quite unexciting BUT… there was a chocolate vending machine right outside my door and this loaded machine made my eyes light up; seeing that machine was the highlight of my day. Can you believe chocolate was the most exciting thing going on in my life at the time? So, I would be at home, studying and I would think 'Which chocolate am I going to have today - Picnic, Kit Kat, Mars Bar or Snickers?' I would tell myself to focus, but pretty soon my mind would be drifting, my thoughts venturing back to the choc-a-block vending machine. 'I could have some chocolate covered nuts or what about that chocolatey wafer biscuit or that gooey nougat caramel.'

"Focus Renae – you have to write this assignment – 2000 words are due on Friday." But… 'Picnic has nuts in it and nuts are healthy and if you have nuts as a snack then you're actually being healthy – that's it, it's a Picnic today.' Surprise, surprise, the chocolate would win every time…. every time. I was good at justifying my reasons why I should have the chocolate. I would tell myself, "you've been so good all day, you went to all your classes, you studied hard, you deserve it;" or "I'll start my new diet on Monday and I may as well have a special treat before the new diet starts." I spent years craving chocolate, resisting, giving in and feeling guilty. The cycle continued and for years I thought I was addicted to chocolate but in the end, after taking a long hard look at the 6 Core Human Needs, I found that I wasn't actually addicted to the chocolate. It was the excitment I was after.

I didn't realise this until my early thirties and I was amazed to find that I could overcome my chocolate addiction by looking at my actual life rather than constantly focusing on not eating the chocolate. So rather than focusing on the food, I started focusing on my life.

Here's what I did exactly:

1. I quit my job and started my own Coaching business – finally working in a field that I am passionate about. Anyone who has ever started a business will know that there is a lot of excitement in getting a business off the ground. But it doesn't stop there – day in, day out there are ups and downs and there is loads of variety. Starting a business is quite the rollercoaster ride. So, I let go, put my hands up and enjoyed the exciting ride and have been doing so ever since.

2. I studied what I wanted to, not what I thought I should. I wanted to finish University. I'd started so I thought I may as well finish; so I decided to make my university days more fun by choosing courses that I was curious and excited about. I did some photography courses, slipped in some creative writing, joined Toastmasters and because I love languages I decided to do a Diploma in Spanish. The Diploma added an extra year to my Degree but I love this language so I didn't mind at all. Besides, four years flew by because I was now having fun, and to top it off, I topped my Spanish class every semester over the entire course, and those grades lifted my Grade Point Average (GPA) and made it sparkle. Much to my surprise, I was placed in the top 5% of my Communications degree. Isn't it interesting what happens when we do things we are actually interested in? We do well, we thrive, we get excited and life becomes more about living and less about existing. Oh, and last but not least…

3. My ex-boyfriend moved out and I was able to sweep up those egg shells that I had been walking on for so long. What was even more fascinating was that my chocolate bar addiction disappeared when I made these changes and at the time of publishing this book, it has been over two and a half years since I have eaten a chocolate bar. This is because I filled

the need of variety in my life using ways that didn't involve chocolate bars. Happy Dance!

3. SIGNIFICANCE

This is the need to feel needed, to feel important, unique and special. This is a need that can escape people and show up without even looking as if it's about emotional eating, but believe me it is. It was ever present in my life.

Some people fill this need by competing with others. Others will fill it by connecting with other human beings, and other people will fill it by tearing others down. I used to fill it with food.

In my past life I worked in Real Estate, in an office full of women and let's just say I was a little bit different. For starters, they were all coffee drinkers and I didn't drink coffee. When they went out to get coffee, they would offer everyone else in the office something except, you guessed it, me. Plus, they were all smokers and on their group cigarette breaks, I would be the one left in the office manning the phones and taking care of reception.

And, maybe it was paranoia setting in but when they came back in I felt they'd been talking about me and that didn't make me feel good at all.

Let's not forget the staff meetings. If they weren't talking over the top of me and I could actually put a suggestion forward, one of the girls would say, "Yeah, that's good but what about this…" making my idea bigger and better, whilst taking all the credit.

So, the way that I gained significance was to take lunch orders for Chinese food and run down the street to collect it. This helped me feel important.

I would be sure to bring back extra spring rolls and prawn chips and I would grab some lollies and chocolates so we had something to snack on in the afternoon. We would joke and laugh as we shared this love of food together. Because I was the provider of the food that people loved so much, I felt important.

But, there was a trade-off. I had to eat rubbish food in order to feel that importance.

Now, for some people who bake treats or birthday cakes for friends, significance could be a need that is lacking in your life; the need to feel needed in this world.

Things have changed significantly for me now. In place of buying Chinese food and chocolate for people in order to gain my significance, I now enjoy the gratitude from my clients for helping them live more abundant and fulfilling lives.

So you can see why it's so important to be doing something that we love, something that we're passionate about, something that makes us want to jump out of bed in the morning and start living on purpose, enjoying some fun hobbies, living out our dreams, making the most of the lives we've been fortunate enough to be given, instead of lying in bed and hitting the snooze button repeatedly.

Yes, it's time to wake up, get up and grab life with two eager hands and fill it up with things that we love! Are you hearing me loud and clear? Live your passion, today. Every day is a blessing. Each and every one of us is here for a significant reason in our significant life. It's time to realise significance isn't about using food in not so constructive ways. Your significance goes so much deeper than that. I read a quote, just before writing this section of the book, that I absolutely love and it has come at the perfect time.

It's from The Motivation Manifesto by Brendon Burchard. "Imagine the end of your life you are standing before your Creator, and He asks: Did you use the time I gifted you each day to be a purposeful being? Did you follow your own path and make your time count? How faithfully did you tend to the dream I sowed in your soul?"

How would you answer?

4. Love and Connection

This is a strong feeling of closeness or union with someone or something. It's the need to be a part of something and be truly connected with another person or group.

I've heard about people suffering from depression that got a dog and in a short amount of time, weren't depressed anymore. People join groups so they can be a part of something that they believe in, and they meet people who are on the same wavelength as them. There's an instant connection with people when you join a club that has people who get you. By being around family who love and accept you, true friends with whom you can really be yourself around or having a partner who you feel really close to, that is what love and connection is about.

So there you have it, the first 4 needs, and remember, if even one of these needs are not being fulfilled in constructive ways, the fulfilment will show up in the form of an addiction, meaning, you will reach for something that is only going to give you short term gratification – such as emotional eating.

We have to fill these needs in constructive ways to have a good life. Once this has been done – Great! Congratulations! It's an incredible achievement! But, why stop there? Why not go one or two steps further and go about getting a great life so you can answer the question 'How are you?' in a true and upbeat way and wholeheartedly mean it.

Rather than answering this question 'How are you?' with: "Not bad," "Ok," or "Can't complain." You can do this - fulfil needs 5 and 6 constructively and that "not bad" could be turned into "Great," "Fantastic," "Super Duper" that will in turn lift the vibe around you, creating an upbeat ripple effect; lifting not only your mood but the mood of others around you. I'm not saying that it is always going to be this way, where every day you are going to be upbeat because the ups and downs in life do happen. I'm also not suggesting that you lie about how you are feeling and say that you are great when you are not feeling that way on a particular day. You are going to have down days; things are not going to go swimmingly all the time but the majority of the time we want to spend happy, right?

We are not here to live a sad existence. We are here to live a happy and fulfilling one.

Let's move on now to see how we can live a life of fulfilment.

5. GROWTH

This is the expansion of capacity, capability or understanding. This is another tricky one, like significance as it can sneak up on you when you don't really know it's happening. Our souls need to grow, and if you've listened to any of the works of Human Behaviour Expert, Dr John DeMartini, you may be familiar with one of his findings. He talks about growth and how our souls crave it and part of this growth is about having small challenges in life, so our souls will constantly seek out challenge. Now, we can either consciously give our souls the challenges we choose, ones that are congruent with our highest values, goals that are inspiring to us that move us forward in the direction we choose to grow or we can choose not to give it those challenges, and not give it challenges that are inspiring to us and if that is case then life, God, the Universe, whatever you choose to call it is going to fill our lives with challenges that are uninspiring to us, such as eating 'addictions'.

So, if you feel your life is one uninspiring challenge after another, which makes it hard for you to get on top of your eating habits, growth could be the need that is lacking in your life, and that means you need to decide now what little challenges you're going to give yourself in order for you to grow in the direction that you choose to grow. If you don't, well, you're definitely going to grow but it will possibly be in your waistline because that's going to be one of the challenges that life throws at you.

So, now, the choice is yours – what challenges are you going to give yourself?

6. Contribution

This is a sense of service and focus on helping, giving to and supporting others. It's the need to give beyond ourselves in a meaningful way. This is a combination of growth and connection as it is giving back to others around us, both individuals and groups. When we have constructively fulfilled our essential needs, we can give to others and still have enough for ourselves. Our giving then becomes selfless as it is with a sense of not wanting anything in return because our other needs have been met in positive ways. Being able to give without expecting anything in return is a beautiful thing and one that is deep within our soul, something we all strive for even if we don't consciously think about doing it as there may be a sense of longing to receive something in return. But, within our core, our very essence, we long to give just to give. When we are truly connected with our spirit and our contribution is without ego that is when we experience our true essence and a deep fulfilment in ourselves and in our lives.

Being able to understand the 6 core human needs and how to fulfil them gives us an insight into our own behaviours and other people's behaviours around us. As these are universal needs, there is no getting around them. We have to fulfil them in one way or another. Either in constructive and fulfilling ways or in unconstructive ways. This can be tricky as there can be a strong pull towards instant gratification (that quick fix) as opposed to meeting our needs in the long-term (long-term happiness). Those unconstructive ways may appear to be serving us when we are acting on them but it is usually about feeding that need in the short-term with short-term gains and momentary satisfaction. If there is no real long-term gain that is taking us towards our goals and leaving us with long-term fulfilment then it is only a way of achieving instant gratification, which, in turn leads to regret and sadness.

Which Unresolved Emotions Are Driving Your Emotional Eating? If you'd like to find out, take our free quiz. You'll find it at:

http://www.overcomeyouremotionaleating.com/

If you discover that you often eat for emotional reasons instead of satisfying your nutritional hunger, then there is a problem. When you obey the urge to eat more than you require, you will gain weight. Excess weight can be more dangerous if you have health conditions such as diabetes, obesity and high blood pressure. It's not only about weight gain however. Personally, I found the main problems with emotional eating was the lack of focus I had in my everyday life, along with low energy, low self-confidence, isolating myself, constantly letting myself down, poor concentration, stomach issues, bloating, water retention and all the negative thoughts and feelings I had around food, and especially after giving into food – the guilt, shame, regret, self-loathing. I'm sure you can name some negative feelings you have too. An emotional roller coaster filled with turmoil on a day to day basis. I was at my wits end when I fortunately came across some new information about how to overcome emotional eating. For two decades I was looking externally for answers and it just wasn't working. I thought I was a failure because I couldn't stick to a diet or control my food intake. I thought I was addicted to food and I hated how weak I (thought I) was. I really was in a terrible place. I felt sad a lot, was frustrated at myself because I couldn't get my act together and most days I felt defeated, like a boxer in a ring who had just taken a massive hit and gone down. It wasn't until I started tuning into my body and listening to what it had to say that I started to make progress. I stopped trying to run from my feelings and started to sit with them, be with them, observe them rather than self-medicate. In my quest for answers I found that there are three main emotions that drive people to emotionally eat. Anger, Sadness and Fear and I would like to share some findings with you.

Let's take a look at Anger first.

ANGER

When I first started doing research on how unresolved emotions drive emotional eating, something that stood out for me was this: 'Anger is one letter short of Danger'. It may not hit you as hard as it hit me but it really made me sit and think about why anger can be so harmful... if suppressed. Thanks to my research, what I went on to realise was that anger in itself is not bad, anger is in fact a very useful emotion... if expressed in constructive ways. It can help motivate and mobilise you into taking positive action.

Anger repression however, can be a whole other story, aside from uncontrolled outbursts (onto innocent bystanders), it can turn into depression and anxiety that we try to deal with through emotionally eating.

It occurred to me that I suppressed anger for years because I thought it was bad. I realised (like a smack in the face) how much of an impact repressing my anger had played a part in my emotional eating. I thought that being angry meant you would be deemed an 'angry bitch'.

This in my opinion was one of the worst things I could imagine; being known as an angry person.

I was brought up thinking that women were beautiful, kind and lovely which is why I acted the way I thought I was supposed to in polite society: polite, sweet, nice, even if I thought or felt differently about what someone said or did. I would be silent if I was not feeling upbeat so that I didn't step out of the expected polite society behaviour. I wouldn't want to make anyone feel uncomfortable or embarrass myself in the process. I wore my mask and although I'm sure that some people could see through my mask at times, at least I wasn't outwardly displaying any negative, violent and turbulent feelings. I felt it just wasn't the right way to behave.

Everything became great, wonderful, and perfect and although I wasn't always feeling upbeat, vibrant and like a winner, my words expressed that I was. It was when I was behind closed doors that I had to really feel, feel the depths of my frustration, the inner resentment that was growing more and more and the regret that I would experience for my action or inaction. So, even though I was feeling all these feelings I didn't know that my lack of expressing my emotions was hindering me from moving forward and stopping me from getting on top of my emotional eating habits.

It wasn't until I met my boyfriend (at a point when I was at my wits end with my emotional eating habits) that I realised I was not saying how I really felt about things and that I was definitely not expressing my true emotions.

I started doing some work with some Coaches and attending personal development seminars and courses and finally began to speak out about myself and what I was really feeling. This was foreign to me because I had never really told anyone how I was feeling. When someone asked: How are you? My reply was great or good thank you (polite society responses). I never told anyone that I felt angry at myself because I'd just eaten a family size block of chocolate and because of that I was so uncomfortably bloated nor would I tell anyone that the tummy tuck I was doing was giving me an extreme belly ache.

I wouldn't tell them that I was so disappointed in myself because I had almost made it through a whole day without having a bag of chips and didn't quite get there (besides, I thought they would never have understood). I kept my true feelings to myself and I let everyone think that I was fine. Besides, they had their own life to worry about, without having to hear about my problems.

I continued to keep my anger, frustration and regret inside. It festered and I suffered quietly.

When I first learnt about expressing anger, I was taken aback. In the first instance I thought I didn't really have it, that I had had some in the past but it had gone away. No biggie – I figured I wouldn't have to take part in the anger exercise because I wasn't feeling angry – I was ok. Just fine, quite peachy. I mean I was smiling so I mustn't have been angry. What, I learnt was that it was healthy to express anger behind the scenes, in a safe environment, either with people you trust or on your own.

What this does is allow you to get anger out in a constructive, non-harmful way so that you are not releasing anger when you are triggered. You choose when you express it instead.

Just so you know what I mean by triggers, take a look at some that you may (or may not) have experienced yourself.

Some examples of triggers:

➲ A car cutting you off (it was their fault, of course) resulting in you verbally abusing someone or flipping the bird (or dishing out another form of angry expression you favour at the time) and you are left fuming, whinging and moaning for hours after the incident. Grrrrrrr!

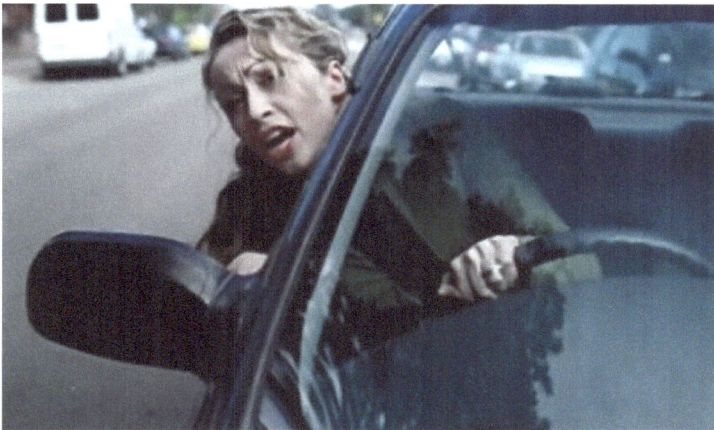

➲ Your partner does something to annoy you… again and you lose it… again and your day or night is spent re-living the argument… again.

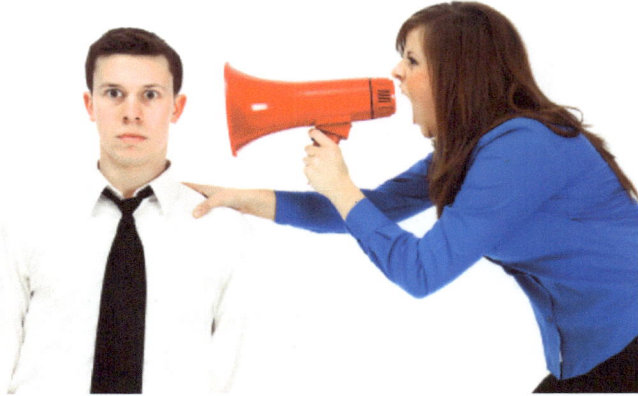

➲ Your boss or a co-worker is being unreasonable; you lose your cool, and regret it afterwards, making it terribly difficult to focus on work or anything else for that matter, when you're not in the right head space.

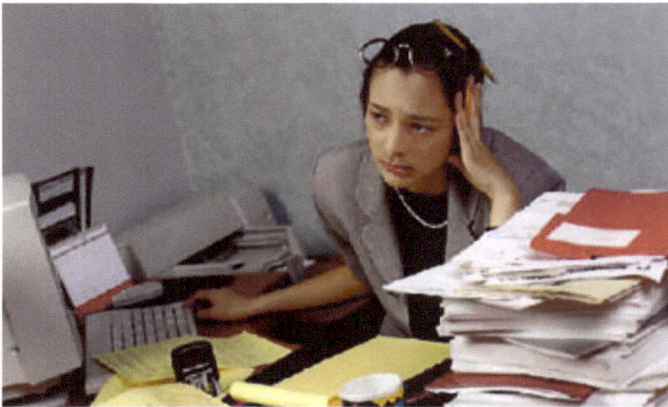

These are all examples of emotional triggers and they occur when we are not in control of our emotions. These reactions can be quite damaging.

So... What's The Best Way to Release Anger?

There are several ways to let anger out behind the scenes. This allows you to empty the tank so that your anger doesn't boil over in a situation that would generally make you angry. This saves you from making a scene, hurting yourself, your reputation and others. It will also help you be more mindful of those strong uncontrollable urges for comfort food you get and give into to console yourself, which in turn make you get even more down on yourself. This happens because you are now dealing with your emotions; listening to them, working with them, rather than stuffing them down with food.

Actor, Will Rogers said, "It takes a lifetime to build a good reputation, but you can lose it in a minute."

This quote should be encouragement enough to do regular anger work.

If you need more of a nudge…. Understand what anger does to you internally – it festers.

Now, who's up for some anger work?

Here are some exercises that can allow you to express your anger in positive ways.

Know that if you have never done any anger work before, it is safe. It's actually safer than not doing anger work as you can choose to do it in a responsive way rather than reacting in a situation that triggers you.

Let the anger work begin!

1. The Punching Bag
   a. It is recommended that you do this in a secure, comfortable space where you won't be disturbed.
   b. One of the best ways to express your anger is with a punching bag and boxing gloves. If you don't have a bag and gloves and are not planning on investing in them, the lounge in your family room and your bare fists can work just as well.

c. Position the punching bag down on the floor and kneel in front of it with your bottom resting on your heels then, put on your boxing gloves.

d. Prepare yourself, taking in a few long deep breaths.

e. Make a fist with one hand, raise yourself off your heels, lift your arm back above your head, opening your chest and hit the punching bag with the side of your fist NOT your knuckles.

f. Be sure to take in a deep breath when you raise and lift your arm back over your head, then let the breath out with force and a big 'Huh' sound as you connect the side of your fist with the punching bag.

g. Change arms and keep alternating from one arm to the next.

h. The first part is just a warm up so go slowly so you avoid injury. The first part should be at about 20% intensity, building up slowly to 40%. Do this for a few minutes. When you feel a little warmer and are ready to increase the intensity, do so. Please pay attention to how you are feeling. Listen to your body so you don't overdo it. Keep increasing your intensity to about 75% for about five minutes.

i. For the last part, give it all you've got; punching into the bag and now turning the big 'HUH' sound into a continuous yell. Bring the sound from your belly so you don't injure your vocal cords. Keep going until you feel you have done enough.

j. When you have finished, sit back and relax, taking in some long deep breaths while you take in the moment.

k. If you live close to your neighbours, E.g. in an apartment, you may want to turn on some music while you do this so you feel more comfortable.

l. It is very important when doing anger work to really give it a good go. Only giving it half your energy is not good enough. Commitment is very important so you can release built up anger and let the anger out. When you punch, be sure to yell, be vocal and let it out. The physical and vocal component work hand in hand so get yelling, release and let go!

m. Note that you don't have to feel angry at the time of the exercise. In fact, I've heard this expression a lot when doing my own anger work in a room full of supportive people; I've even said it myself as I mentioned earlier. "I don't feel angry at the moment." The whole point of anger work is to be proactive with the emotion as opposed to reacting when anger hits.

n. Start releasing and letting loose and anger will come to the surface with your participation.

SADNESS

Human beings are emotional beings. There is no tiptoeing around it. No matter how much we don't want to feel the 'negative' feelings, we are going to have to at some point. We mess up sometimes which brings us down, we hurt ourselves, we hurt others (whether it's intentional or not) and people that we love and care for pass away. There is no getting around this. One way or another we are going to feel sadness at some point in our lives. It's inevitable. This is why it is so important to condition ourselves.

Physically: keeping our body strong.

Mentally: keeping our mind sharp.

Emotionally: being in control of our emotions so we are not triggered.

Crying is extremely healing. When it is done properly it is therapeutic. The problem is that a lot of the time when we cry, we feel ashamed and stop the flow of tears before the cry has finished, meaning we only release a small amount of the tears that were there so there is still a build-up. You know you've had a good cry when you exhale at the end. The sigh is your way of knowing that there's been a great release of built up emotions.

A way I like to think about our emotions is by thinking that every emotion builds up in its very own tank.

For example: The Sadness Tank – because we judge sadness as a negative emotion, we cut it off and by doing this we end up storing it. The more we bottle it up, the more it builds, until one day it overflows and there is no choice but to release it when there is no more room to store it.

To prevent the overflow and the outbursts, we need to learn how to express our sadness when we choose and let the tears flow until we are physically spent. By doing this and having a good cry at a time and place of our choosing will help us heal and give us back control of our emotions.

You could put on a sad movie or read a letter that triggers your sadness. However you choose to express sadness is up to you. It's time to heal. Anything is better than leaving it to build up inside of you.

Emotion is energy in motion. This means, the energy moves, it needs to move. If it doesn't, if it gets suppressed, it gets stuck, builds up and creates pressure in the body. Eventually that pressure has to release, meaning the place of least resistance in your body will be affected. Maybe there is a history of heart disease in your family, or there could be an imbalance in one area of your body. That area could be where your body lets go.

Working with your sadness will keep the energy flowing and releasing.

When the sadness has passed, it creates a better flow of energy in your body and you will be able to move forward: cleaner, clearer and with more vitality.

What would you do better once your sadness has been released?

Fear

This is a massive driver.... That's what's going to get you moving.

Now let's take the emotion of fear and zoom in on when an emotional eater is living in fear.

Fear is a valuable emotion, like any other. Our bodies will naturally respond with fear when there is a perceived threat. We must not think of fear as a bad emotion overall. Fear is legitimate feedback. It has kept us safe time and time again (especially throughout our childhood, when we didn't have much experience in the world... when we needed it most). It stopped us from carelessly crossing the road when there was oncoming traffic (thanks to our parents' guidance), it kept our little hands away from the stovetop, prevented us from breaking the law or jumping off the roof with a superman cape on.

Fear has served us well in the past and will continue to serve us well in the future... if we respond to it in a situation that will help and not hinder us.

If, however, we let (irrational) fear take us over, it can control our thoughts, our words and our actions and therefore prevent us from living an extraordinary and pro-active life.

Are you really living or merely existing?

Do you get up out of bed every morning pumped because you have another day to devour, with new and exciting challenges?

Or, do you find yourself crawling out of bed unmotivated and lethargic because 'it's just another day?'

And, does the expression 'Same '#hit' different day.' cross your mind regularly?

If the last two questions resonate with you then your emotional eating could very well be driven by fear.

Fear activates our fight or flight response which was highly necessary for us as children (as we were new in the world and had to learn our way around) and for our ancestors when there were real dangers such as fleeing from a hungry lion (or in the case of pro-surfer Mick

Fanning's shark encounter… where he fought off the hungry animal with his bare hands), but in this day and age, now that we have learnt what to stay away from for our safety, we need to learn how to step into our fear so we can turn it into power.

I have spoken to hundreds of people on the topic of fear and what prevents them from living the life they really want. What continually comes up is:

'I don't have the confidence'.

People think they lack confidence and that is why they are not living the life they so desire. Well, let me tell you something, it's not confidence you lack. It's courage.

You gain confidence by doing things… you just have to have the courage to start.

By having the courage to step into your fear, you will realise how much courage you really have.

Your fear is the doorway to world of truth, you just have to open the door and put one foot in front of the other.

Another way we can look at fear is through the

PAIN – PLEASURE model.

Note that PAIN can be substituted with FEAR and PLEASURE can be substituted with LOVE.

The reason for this is because everything we do in our lives is to Avoid Pain or Get Pleasure. The same goes for Fear and Love as we are constantly trying to get away from fear and go towards love.

So in terms of the PAIN – PLEASURE model, pleasure is the goal. And, what we really want is for our pleasure to last. We want the long-term pleasure that is going to take some time to achieve but don't want to go through the pain to achieve it.

Pleasure in the near future is the quickest pleasure to achieve. (Emotional eaters will get this short-term pleasure from food). It's momentary satisfaction, the nearest and most instant pleasure.

Eg. You want to lose weight (but your feelings are getting uncomfortable) and you have gone a day or two without having a chocolate. The fear of this pain in the now (dealing with your emotions rather than having a quick fix that you normally get through chocolate) stops you from getting to the distant future pleasure because you question if you will survive the pain.

The Pleasure Pain Model

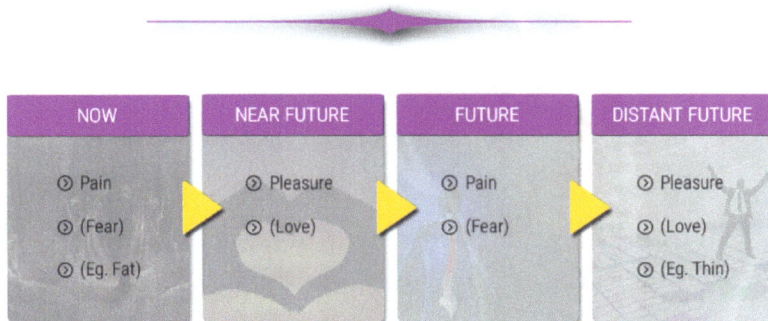

NOW	NEAR FUTURE	FUTURE	DISTANT FUTURE
⊙ Pain	⊙ Pleasure	⊙ Pain	⊙ Pleasure
⊙ (Fear)	⊙ (Love)	⊙ (Fear)	⊙ (Love)
⊙ (Eg. Fat)			⊙ (Eg. Thin)

Emotional eaters want instant pleasure. That instant gratification, that quick fix. They want to avoid pain and eating the chocolate is how they do this.

The truth of the matter is that you are in pain now – your current pain is home to you; you are comfortable in this pain.

It's the fear (pain) of the unknown that stops people from getting what they really want because the fear (pain) of the unknown is the biggest fear in the human psyche. We think we won't survive it.

It was my reality for years.

It is when we are extremely fed up, have our backs against the wall, when we hit rock bottom or it comes down to a matter of life or death we are more likely to say, 'That's It,' 'I'm going to get on top of my eating habits', because we are sick and tired of being sick and tired. This happens when THE FEAR OF WHAT YOUR LIFE WILL LOOK LIKE IF YOU DON'T DO SOMETHING THAT

TAKES YOU IN THE OTHER DIRECTION takes hold. What's interesting is that FEAR is still the driver but it's the fear of not wanting to settle for mediocre or even less than mediocre anymore. It's the fear of what it's going to cost you if you don't take action. Focus on that to mobilise you. Focus on that when you are embracing uncomfortable emotions. By shifting your focus to the pain of inactivity (staying the same) and writing down what that will cost you in 1 year, 5 years, 10 years and so on, that's what's going to get you moving in the direction of your long-term pleasure.

Exercise: What's it going to cost you in 1 year, 5 years and even 10 years if nothing around the subject of your emotional eating changes?

Write your findings in your journal. If your journal is not handy at the moment, jot down some notes below and elaborate on them when you have your journal at the ready:

_____

_____

_____

_____

_____

_____

_____

_____

_____

_____

_____

_____

_____

_____

Once you've looked at what it's going to cost you if you stay the same, start looking at the pleasure of taking action to move you forward.

What will it give you when you take action and start moving forward?

_____

_____

_____

_____

_____

_____

_____

_____

_____

_____

_____

_____

_____

_____

Another thing that keeps people on track is progress. When you notice changes, say you lose two kilos in the first week of your weight loss journey – you get excited and see that what you are doing is working for you. Making sure you map out your progress, being sure to write down what you have achieved will keep you going towards your goals and towards the pleasure that you envision in the future.

To continue on this path to your future goals you must know why it is so important to reach your goals. Why do you want a life free from emotional eating? Know your real driver that is taking you away from pain and towards long-term pleasure. What are you really hungry for?

What's your why?

_____

_____

_____

_____

_____

_____

_____

_____

_____

_____

_____

_____

_____

_____

When you know your why – it's time to set yourself up for success. But first, if you haven't done so already, take our free quiz to see which unresolved emotions are driving your emotional eating:

http://www.overcomeyouremotionaleating.com/

What can I do to set myself up for success?

When it comes to success, it is up to you. No one is going to do the work for you. You have to be dedicated to making yourself a better person and dedicated to continuously going after what it is you really want. That means devoting your time and your energy to your cause. If you are willing to invest in yourself and willing to back yourself one hundred per cent, you will get the results you deserve.

There are many ways you can set yourself up for success. I'm sharing four sure-fire, tried and tested ways to get you on the path of overcoming emotional eating and on your way to living an extraordinary life.

Find a mentor – someone who has been successful in achieving what you want to achieve. They will help you get to where you want to go quicker than if you were to go at it alone.

Believe in yourself – this is a massive factor in you getting to your destination. This may mean you have to change your beliefs if your old ones don't serve you anymore. How cool is that – you can actually choose your beliefs so they empower you! When you believe, the obstacles are less challenging because you can see the reward, there is no denying it – you are there and it's only a matter of time before your body catches up.

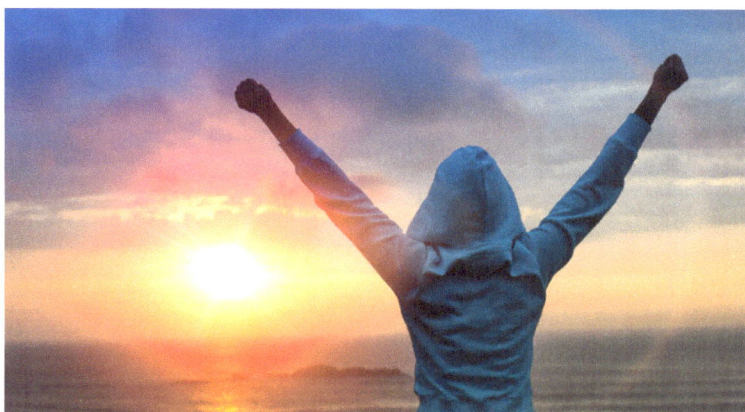

Take Action – do something every day that will take you closer to your goal. Be consistent. Your action will get you your results and your results will reinforce your belief in yourself as you have solid proof that you are achieving your goal.

Strengthen your mind – visualise yourself when you've reached your goal, create a vision board and look at it daily, say affirmations – do whatever it takes to condition your mind. By doing these things daily, there is no question that you will be where you want to be. Empowered, Strong, Inspired and Inspiring.

YOUR HIGHEST VALUES

Our values are a calling from our heart, not from our head. They are what we truly desire to do, not what we think we should do. They are our real, heart-felt why behind what we do or want to do in life. When you identify your values in life, you learn how to create greater happiness, cope better with stress, experience improved performance etc. If you choose to live by your values every day, you will enjoy life to the fullest.

When did you last experience happiness and what was driving that happiness? Consider your personal life and your work experiences. You may have been happiest at work or even and more likely when doing something you like best.

A survey conducted by Open Universities in Australia showed that approximately 7.4 million of Australia's 11.5 million workers are not happy in their current job. And just under half of the nation's workers admit they got into their present career by "falling into it."

These are scary statistics yet sadly, not surprising. Many people simply go through the motions and do what they have to do, unconsciously. A big part of this comes down to not knowing your values. A large number of people simply do not know their values and how can you live to your values if you don't know them?

Despite the grim facts, there are a rising number of people who are waking up and choosing to live a life on their terms. An ever growing number of entrepreneurs for example, creating their dream life, giving up the stability of their 9 to 5 and taking matters into their own hands in an attempt to live the life they were born to. More and more people are choosing to do what they love to do, following their passion and making their time on this earth really count.

Author, Bonnie Ware worked in palliative care and while spending time with patients who were coming to the end of their life, she discovered some common themes amongst them and felt it was important to share this information. Bonnie went on to write a book entitled 'The Top Five Regrets of the Dying.' The biggest regret expressed was "I wish I'd had the courage to live a life true to myself, not the life others expected of me."

We do, do, do, every day, after day, after day and so much of what we are doing is not filling us up. A lot of what we do is just so we can get it done and it really gets us down.

If you are one of the fortunate ones who firstly, knows your top five values and can then go on to say that you are truly living life by your highest values, I take my hat off to you. That, my friend is fantastic! (Not that my approval is any consolation) What's true though is this, life is meant to be lived and lived well. Happy. Free. In love... with how you have chosen to pass your time and who you have chosen to pass your time with in this extraordinary universe.

If you are not quite sure of your values as yet and find yourself asking 'Is this all there is?' It may be time to check in with what your heart's calling is and what you really want to be doing in life, starting with finding your values and then, living to them.

The best way to determine your values is through a series of questions. In 'The Values Factor' by Human Behavior expert Dr John Demartini, there are a series of questions that will help you determine your highest values. Take some time to answer them, below.

Answer the questions (with 3 answers each) to find out what your top 5 highest values are.

1. *What items do you fill your home or working space with?*
   We usually keep things that are important to us around us so we can see them. If there are items that are stashed away and have been for some time, they may not mean as much to you as you think they do.

Take a look around your home and your place of work – what do you see?

a) _____

b) _____

c) _____

2. *How do you choose to pass your time?*
   Have you ever let the sentence "I don't have enough time to do what I love" pass your lips? Has it been on several occasions? I'm sorry to break this news to you; we do what is most important to us, for whatever reason, we make the choice to do what we value most.

Which three ways do you spend most of your time?

a) _____

b) _____

c) _____

3. *How do you use your precious energy?*
   We spend our energy on things that are inspiring to us. Things that drain us are things that we don't find in the list of our highest values. Our energy is precious, as it runs out we realise this more. It is to be spent wisely, doing things that we are passionate about. It is a fact that when we do something that we truly value, we are left with more energy than when we began. When we do what we love and love what we do, the world is a better place.

Which actions do you spend your precious energy on?

a) _____

b) _____

c) _____

4. *What do you spend your money on?*

We spend money on things that matter to us most. Things we don't value and don't see value in makes us want to hang onto our cash. A parent may see value in their child's education and so, sends them to a private school. Another parent may value travel more than education so the money they save on private school fees allows them to take their family on a yearly holiday overseas.

Name three items you spend your money on most:

a) _____

b) _____

c) _____

5. *In which areas of your life are you most organised?*

There is order in the areas of our lives that we truly value and disorder in the areas that are low on our list of values. Where do you have the most order and organisation? Some examples are your house, your work space, health and wellbeing, your wardrobe, your business and the way you conduct it, your study regime and your spiritual practice. There will be an area of your life that you keep organised most.

List three areas or items that you have most organised:

a) _____

b) _____

c) _____

6. *In which areas of your life are you most reliable & disciplined?*
   When I was younger I was always told to practice my guitar but it wasn't one of my highest values when I was a kid. All I wanted to do was play with my friends or my dolls. When we truly value something we don't need to be told or reminded to do it. Our want to do it, speak about it, learn about it comes from a deep longing from within. Where are you most focused? In which aspects of your life are you most reliable? Think about your relationships, the activities you take part in and the goals that you set for yourself.

   Name three activities you are most reliable and focused:

a) _____

b) _____

c) _____

7. *What occupies your thoughts most?*
   Let's forget about any negative thoughts you may have, along with fantasies or those pesky 'shoulds' or 'should haves'. These thoughts are about what we want in our lives, how we want our lives to be and what we are making happen.

   Name the three thoughts that you have most that you are bringing to reality:

a) _____

b) _____

c) _____

8. *What do you find yourself visualising the most that is becoming a reality?*

   We are talking truth here, not fantasies. What do you visualise in your life that you are making happen? In Dr Demartini's case he visualises travelling the world, I'm talking the whole world and going to every country and teaching people. This is what he visualises and is making happen.

   Now it's your turn, which results are you visualising and making happen?

a) _____

b) _____

c) _____

9. *What comes up in your internal dialogue?*

   What do you find you talk to yourself about most? We are not speaking about any negative self-talk in this case. We are speaking about the internal dialogue that you use to communicate with yourself about your desires, things that you want to happen that you are actually making happen.

   Name three things you most often talk to yourself about, outcomes that you want and are making happen in your life:

a) _____

b) _____

c) _____

10. In social situations, what do you speak about?

There are topics that can get us talking for hours, topics that we can keep speaking about until the cows come home. What do you find yourself asking people regularly? Are there subjects that you find yourself bringing consistently into a conversation? It is easy to figure out other people's values by the questions they ask. If they speak a lot about children, it shows that children, either theirs or yours mean something to them. If they ask what you've been cooking lately, then cooking means something to them.

Fill in the blanks with three topics you find yourself speaking to people about:

a) _____

b) _____

c) _____

11. What inspires you most?

What excites you? What really wakes you up and gets your blood pumping? What lights your eyes up? This doesn't have to only revolve around 'what', it could be a person. Who inspires you? Who do you love to be around? Who would you love to be around? What traits do people that inspire you have?

Jot down three things, actions, people or results that inspire you – think about what is common in all of them:

a) _____

b) _____

c) _____

12. *What goals have you set that you are bringing to fruition?*

We are speaking about goals that you are consistently taking action on so you can turn them into a reality. Dreams remain dreams unless we take action and turn them into something that we would love to bring about. There is no fantasy in this question – this is something that you have been making happen and one step at a time with dedication and persistence are creating right before your very eyes.

Write down three goals that you've been creating on a consistent basis:

a) _____

b) _____

c) _____

13. *Which topics do you love to learn most about?*

Think about which section of the Newsagency, library or bookstore you head to when you enter. Which TV shows do you watch? Are there documentaries that you prefer to watch over others? Do you find yourself looking into topics so you can get more information?

Name three things you enjoy reading about or studying:

a) _____

b) _____

c) _____

Now that you've completed the questions, you'll see that there is some repetition in your answers. Look at the symmetry. For example: Having a drink with friends, going out to dinner with like-minded people. Watch out for the patterns. Note how many times your answers are repeated and put them in order of 1st, 2nd, 3rd, 4th and 5th. This will give you a good indication of what your highest values are.

Your values will show you what is most important in your life and you can start building your dream life around these values.

Write your values here:

_____

_____

_____

_____

_____

_____

_____

_____

_____

_____

So here are your values, this doesn't mean that this is final as you can reshape your values and change the order of them as you like – just like anything – where there is a will there is a way, however this will give you awareness of what your values are at present and help you create a life that is on purpose instead of just plodding along and watching time pass you by.

OVERCOMING BULIMIA

There was something deep within me that was screaming out to stop this insanity once and for all. I was working on myself, learning more about who I am and liking what I found. I was showing up, making a decision every day to choose my own personal freedom. I was sick of my life as I knew it and I was doing everything to take me towards change, something better, a new way of living. I had thought time and time again about giving up on bulimia and although I had heard some nightmare stories from other sufferers; from throwing up blood to excessive tooth cavities that make it impossible for sufferers to chew hard food, ripped oesophagus, acid reflux, cardiac arrest, so many damaging consequences, the thing that scared me most was the possibility of gaining weight because I didn't know how to control my eating habits. Bulimia was like my get out of jail free card. I thought I could eat whatever I wanted, whenever I wanted and not gain weight, besides, nobody knew about it. It was even easier when I lived alone or shared a place with people that were on a different schedule to me and hardly ever home when I was. I was free to do whatever I liked and I was able to keep my mask on, carry on with my act and now my cover would be blown because I thought I would put on weight... people would know that something was wrong.

After all the self-inflicted abuse though, I think I'm one of the lucky ones because I have come out the other side stronger than I imagined. Aside from the abuse I did to my body for so many years, I've come out alive and driven with a passion to help others overcome emotional eating. I have no regrets now around what I have been through, yes my life would've been different if I'd had control over what I ate throughout the years, but this is the path I have chosen and I feel that it is my calling now to work with other men and women to help them find their freedom, this freedom that I now enjoy. I never thought that I would be free of over-eating; I never thought I could give up chocolate bars. I never thought I could have complete control over what I ate. You might be reading this now and think you can't either. I'm sure you've heard people say time and time again; 'If I can, you can.' Well it's true. I really mean it when I say, 'If I can beat emotional eating, you can too.' I have no doubt about that. I believe in you.

Never in a million years did I think I could go to the movies without getting a choc top or leave the house without a packet of chips in my bag. I had tried time and time again to stop the vicious cycle but to no avail. I thought I was going to be going through bouts of abuse, binging, purging, restriction and diets for the rest of my life. I thought that was my way, but now I know there is another way, a way that works from the inside out, a way that looks at the cause of why we are driven to emotionally eat, rather than focusing on the symptoms - all that surface stuff, the surface stuff that only seems to work for a short period of time.

When I was in my early thirties and met my incredible boyfriend, someone who loved me just the way I am, with total acceptance and no judgement, I felt that it was time to come clean and fess up about what I did behind closed doors, let him know who I really was. I knew I was in safe company and able to share something that deep down I wanted to stop but didn't believe I could without support. I thought that if I told someone who I trusted, someone I could confide in, I would be able to beat this. It was a difficult decision, because I knew that once I confessed, there was no turning back. It took some time for me to come clean and be real, I remember building it up so much that I could barely say the words but when I did, my boyfriend replied: "So?" I couldn't believe his reaction, I mean this was a big deal and all he could say was "So." He told me that it wasn't that bad, it wasn't a big deal and I could beat it. I was shocked. He didn't think I was any less of a person, any less of a girlfriend or any less perfect than what he knew me to be.

Telling someone who believed in me and who loved me for who I am was the first step to recovery. Admitting there was a problem was the first step to freedom. Now, that I had a problem, a problem that I was willing to acknowledge and admit to, I could go about creating a solution. I was frightened though, because I knew I had to do this now as I was no longer on my own and my progress would be shared. This one confession led to a chain of events that would take me forward to where I wanted to go. To recovery.

I ended up in the 'Beyond Success' coaching program with the intention of becoming a Coach. I was very excited about this because not only did I get to train under and learn from my inspiring Mentors: Paul & Mary Blackburn, I got my own Master Coach in this program, a Coach that I could confide in and tell things that I had never told to anyone. Steph was firstly there to help me sort out my inner turmoil and secondly, to help me learn how to become a qualified Coach.

I wasn't forthcoming with my "secrets" right from the start, it took me some time to confide in my Coach and although everything I said was received without judgment from her, I was still very afraid. There was always an element of mistrust that I held in people because, goodness forbid, my secrets would be out and I would be judged by the world 'as if my stuff is the most important stuff in the world' and 'as if there aren't others that have the same issues as me.' I learnt to trust my Coach and trust myself. It was so refreshing to let go of the thought that I was constantly being judged. What unfolded was a discovery that I was the one that had been judging myself all this time, much to my surprise. It had been me that had been labelling myself, it had been me that had been calling myself fat, it had been me that allowed that judgement to expand and fester. It was me all along. And so I thought, if it had been me judging myself all along, surely I could change this situation and make it positive?

My Coach was an incredible support and I am so grateful to her for the hours that she listened to me intently, the hours she accepted me wholeheartedly and the hours of her time that she gave me. It helped, more than she could know, it helped me let go of my judgment and embrace my love for myself and my love and gratitude for Coaching. Coaching has given me purpose and it's made me step into my power and what's more, it has helped me let go of constant self-judgment, that inner voice telling me that I'm not good enough and most importantly, it's helped me let go of Bulimia. As I write I am over five years free of Bulimia and it is such an incredible feeling. I feel free and that freedom has given me the push to write this book releasing a story that I held so tightly, a story that I didn't want to share because of the fear of judgment. I now feel empowered sharing my story and if it helps other men and women free themselves from the clutches that food has over them then this whole journey has been worth it.

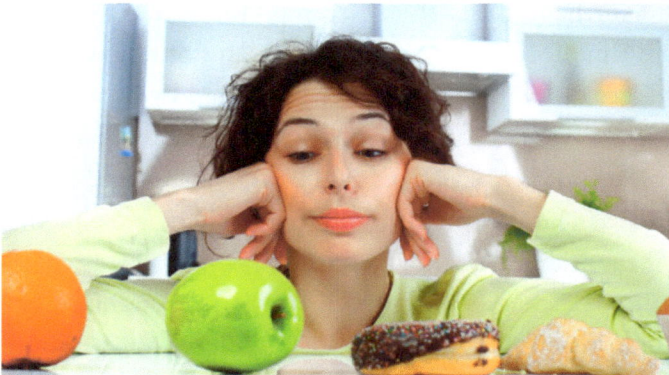

Chapter Four

OVERCOMING EMOTIONAL EATING

It was one thing to give up on Bulimia and it was another to take control of my eating habits and be in complete control of what I ate. I had to go where I hadn't gone before. I had to get to know myself. I had to look inside and go on a journey with the relationship I had with food. So, I would sit with myself, every day. I made it a non-negotiable to sit with myself and be an observer without judgement to what was happening in my body. An itch would come up and I wouldn't scratch it, I would just be there with it and witness it change and in minutes it would pass as if the itch never existed. I would feel sensations throughout my body, be present with them and observe how they passed. I learnt that emotions are energy in motion. They come and go, rise and fall, dance and tumble and by eating when I wasn't hungry I was:

1. Not able to witness them and see the beauty of who I, who we as human beings really are.

And

2. Numbing and suppressing my emotions; bolting from them at the first glimpse of discomfort.

I learnt that when I overate I was not listening to what my body or soul wanted; when I overate I was listening to what my mind or ego wanted. The mind wants us to change the channel because it doesn't want us to tune into our heart's desires. It wants instant satisfaction which means it will always be seeking external sources to make it happy... this is not long-lasting nor true happiness. The mind is about thinking, not feeling and logic doesn't cut it when it comes to emotional eating. Tuning into our emotions is what's going to help us understand what we really want and who we really are. The clue is in the title... Emotional Eating. That means there is a doorway behind that clue and I had to enter it and look around. It's scary at first because it's new and completely different to what I grew up believing. Sitting with your emotions is not something we were taught to do in school, nor was I ever taught this at home. Tuning in requires staying still, sitting through the boredom, the discomfort and the fear that emotional eaters normally try to numb with food, whether consciously or unconsciously. It means breathing, arriving in our body, getting grounded by noticing our surroundings, feeling the ground below us and being grateful for our body and everything it has done and continues to do for us.

I had to learn to love myself again because that was the only way I was going to move forward. I had to stop the short term search for satisfaction: running away from my emotions through food and instead tune in. I had to stop dieting as it only led to binging, restriction that led to starving myself and yep, you guessed it overeating. I had to try something that I hadn't tried before. Emotional eating constantly left me feeling empty and I was always one more bite away from momentary satisfaction. Dieting left me feeling guilty because I would always break the diet (and start again on Monday) and beat myself up in the process and restriction would leave me feeling deprived. Let me just zoom in on what I just said. All the ways I repeatedly tried to combat emotional eating left me feeling empty, guilty and deprived. This is why focusing on the symptoms to combat emotional eating does not work. It doesn't work because that strategy is built on negativity: fear, guilt, deprivation, shame, judgment, self-loathing and lack of trust in self. We cannot build a strong, loving, honest, long-term, open relationship with ourselves if we constantly abuse and punish ourselves.

Self-hatred doesn't lead to love. Shaming doesn't lead to love. Starvation doesn't lead to love. If you starve yourself through food, you end up a starved person. So, what leads to love and loving yourself? Love does. Love leads to love. I had to learn to love myself and learn how to do that through my relationship with food. That was my doorway. I had to turn on my curiosity and get interested in what I was doing and why I was doing it. My relationship with food was here to teach me a lesson.

Have you heard the Buddhist proverb "When the student is ready the teacher will appear?" Well I was ready and my relationship with food was my teacher and a fantastic teacher at that. I learnt so much about myself and why I do what I do. I learnt so much about mindfulness and awareness and I loved the simplicity of my findings. Life is simple; it is us that complicate it. Getting to know myself was one of the most beautiful things I could ever have done. It has not only brought me more fulfillment in my life, it has filled me with so much joy, love, compassion and gratitude for myself and because my tank is full of the good stuff, I can now share that with others. This whole experience has given me an understanding of what I really want out of life and how I want to live my life. It has given me purpose.

It is with a light heart that I write this because I feel Free at last, Free at last, thank God almighty, I'm free at last!

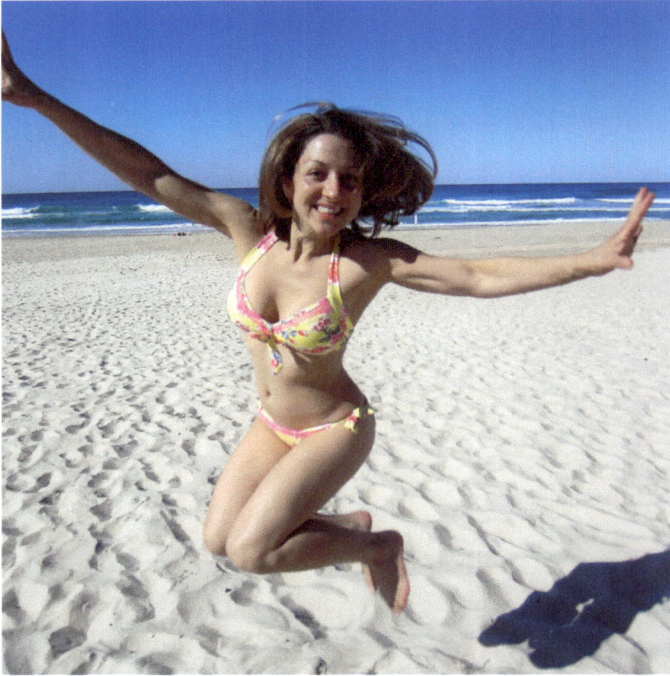

About the Author

Renae was an emotional eater from a very early age. She was just a small child when she found herself constantly eating for reasons other than hunger. If she wasn't eating she was either thinking about her next meal or regretting her last one. Renae would overeat, binge and purge and struggled with the vicious emotional eating cycle right throughout her adolescence, all throughout her twenties and into her early thirties. After years of struggling with food, Renae is now ecstatic to be free from Emotional Eating and Bulimia and is on a mission to help other people, both men and women to free themselves from self-sabotage. Renae knows first-hand what it's like to be an emotional eater – It's very painful – there is a lot of guilt, shame and constant beatings from self about the food consumed along with poor self-image and because of this Renae isolated herself a lot growing up.

While studying her Marketing degree Renae became a Coach and it led her to understand the messages that Marketers put out there to make us want to eat all the 'good' stuff, which is great at the time but that momentary satisfaction doesn't last and we end up on a continuous vicious cycle of blame, guilt, regret and self-hatred. From Renae's research, she realised that emotional eating is not a person's fault; it doesn't come down to lack of willpower or just because a person loves a certain food. It goes deeper than that. Renae has found that too many people are addressing the symptoms with diets and meal plans instead of addressing the cause. Renae says "It's time we hone in on the cause, the root of why we reach for certain foods at certain times." People need to understand their driver so they can overcome emotional eating for good. It's about working from the inside out, not the outside in.

If you'd like to get started on your 'Overcome Your Emotional Eating' journey, please visit:

http://www.overcomeyouremotionaleating.com/

'My Best Friend Was The Chocolate Cake' is Renae's first book. Renae is currently working on her second book around the same topic which also happens to be one of her favourite topics *'Overcoming Emotional Eating'.*

If you would like to be kept in the loop about Renae's upcoming book, get in touch just to chat or if you'd like to learn more about Renae's 12-week online program, you can contact her at

http://www.overcomeyouremotionaleating.com/contact/

BIBLIOGRAPHY

*

http://www.overcomeyouremotionaleating.com/references/

www.ingramcontent.com/pod-product-compliance
Lightning Source LLC
Chambersburg PA
CBHW041217270326
41931CB00001B/8